5 minute core routines for seniors

28 day challenge with simple exercise to boost balance, lose weight and flexibility for healthy aging

Patrick C. Lau

TABLE OF CONTENT

Dear Reader,

Thank you for choosing 5 minute core routines for seniors ;28-Day Challenge with Simple exercise to Boost Balance, lose weight and Flexibility for Healthy Aging. Your decision to explore and improve your health is truly commendable, and I am honored that you have selected this book to assist in the pursuit of a healthy and proper aging.

This book has been carefully crafted to ensure that the content is both accessible and effective for seniors, promoting a healthier and more active lifestyle.

Thank you once again for your trust and support. I hope you find this book to be a valuable companion in your pursuit of a healthier and more active life.

WHY YOU NEED THIS BOOK

Our bodies evolve, bringing with them new obstacles such as stiffness, diminished mobility, and an increased chance of falling. However, growing older does not imply losing strength, agility, or confidence. This is where the book comes into its own.

Reclaim Your Vitality

This book is written exclusively for seniors, addressing the unique demands and limits that come with age. It provides a thorough 28-day regimen that integrates effortlessly into your regular routine, taking only five minutes per day. These exercises are not only basic but very effective at targeting the core muscles, which are essential for maintaining balance and flexibility.

Improve Balance And Prevent Falls

Falls are the biggest cause of injury among elderly. Strengthening your core can help to lessen this risk by increasing balance and stability. The workouts in this book are designed to improve these qualities, allowing you to walk confidently while lessening your fear of falling.

Enhance Flexibility and Mobility

As we become older, we often experience stiffness and limited flexibility. This book contains exercises that gently stretch and strengthen your muscles, so extending your range of motion and making daily tasks easier and more pleasant. Imagine being able to bend, reach, and rotate freely again.

Boost Confidence And Independence

Feeling powerful and steady boosts your confidence. By devoting only five minutes every day to these workouts, you'll see a significant increase in your physical ability. This increase in confidence can improve your overall quality of life, allowing you to keep your freedom and participate in activities that you like.

Easy To Follow

Each activity in this book has clear directions, making it simple to follow along. Whether you're new to exercise or searching for a safe method to keep active, these routines are intended to be simple and achievable for everyone.

A Commitment To Your Health

Investing in your health is the greatest present you can offer yourself. This 28-day challenge is an effort to improve your well-being one step at a time. It's never too late to begin, and the results will be well worth the effort.

A Supportive Guide

This book is more than simply a compilation of exercises; it's a helpful companion on your path to better aging. It provides motivational thoughts and practical guidance to help you stay engaged and makes the most of each day.

Who is the book for?

The program 5 minute core routines for senior 28 -day challenge with simple exercise to boost balance and flexibility for healthy aging is intended for seniors who want to improve their physical health and quality of life. This book is intended for

1. **Seniors Seeking Enhanced Mobility**: This book offers simple activities to increase balance and flexibility, making it easy to include into your everyday routine. The workouts are particularly designed to meet the needs of seniors, ensuring that they are safe, effective, and accessible to all fitness levels.

2. **Those New to Exercise:** If you haven't exercised in a while or are new to working out, don't worry. This book is perfect for beginners. The routines are simple and designed to gradually build your

strength and confidence, making it easy to start and stick with a regular exercise program.

3. **Active Seniors Looking to Maintain Fitness:** For those who already have an active lifestyle, this book offers a convenient way to incorporate quick, effective core exercises into your routine. The 5-minute sessions are a great addition to your existing activities, helping to maintain and enhance your current fitness level.

4. **Individuals Recovering from Injury or Illness:** If you're recovering from an injury or illness and need gentle exercises to regain strength and mobility, these routines are ideal. They are designed to be low-impact and can be adjusted to suit your current abilities and needs.

5. **Caregivers and Family Members:** This book is also a valuable resource for caregivers and family members looking to support the health and well-being of their senior loved ones. The exercises can

be done together, encouraging a sense of community and shared commitment to healthy aging.

6. **Anyone Interested in Aging Gracefully:** Aging is a natural part of life, and staying active is key to aging gracefully. Whether you're looking to improve your physical health, enhance your balance, or simply stay active and independent, this book offers a practical and enjoyable way to achieve your goals.

No matter your current fitness level or experience, 5 minute core routines for senior is here to help you take control of your health, boost your confidence, and embrace a more active, fulfilling lifestyle. Join us on this 28-day journey and discover the benefits of simple, daily routines that can transform your life.

Who Else Can Benefit?

While this book is primarily designed for seniors, the benefits of 5 minute core routines for senior extend far beyond this group. These simple yet effective routines can be a valuable addition to the fitness regimen of various individuals. Here's a look at who else can benefit from these exercises:

1. Busy Professionals:

In the hustle and bustle of daily life, making out time for exercise can be difficult. Busy professionals, juggling work and personal commitments, often struggle to incorporate fitness into their routines. These 5-minute exercises offer a quick and efficient solution, allowing them to maintain core strength and flexibility without a significant time investment.

2. New Parents

For new parents, time is a precious commodity. Between caring for a newborn and managing household tasks, dedicating time to personal fitness can seem impossible. These short, manageable exercises can help new parents stay active and healthy, setting a positive example for their growing families.

3. Individuals Recovering from Injury

People recovering from injuries often need gentle, low-impact exercises to regain strength and mobility. The routines in this book are designed to be safe and accessible, making them ideal for those in the rehabilitation phase. Always consult with a healthcare professional before starting any new exercise program during recovery.

4. Fitness Beginners

Starting a new fitness journey can be daunting for beginners. The simplicity and brevity of these 5-minute routines make them an excellent starting point for anyone new to exercise. They help build a foundation of core strength and balance, encouraging confidence and consistency in physical activity.

5. Active Older Adults

Even older adults who are already active can benefit from these core exercises. Incorporating these routines into their existing fitness strategy can enhance their overall strength, balance, and flexibility, contributing to better performance in other physical activities and everyday tasks.

6. Individuals with Sedentary Lifestyles

Those with sedentary lifestyles, often due to desk jobs or prolonged periods of inactivity, can experience significant improvements in their physical well-being by integrating these exercises. Strengthening the core can alleviate back pain, improve posture, and counteract the negative effects of prolonged sitting.

7. Caregivers

Caregivers, whether professionals or family members, often put others' needs before their own, leading to neglect of their own health, these quick and easy exercises can be a convenient way for caregivers to maintain their strength and flexibility, ensuring they stay healthy and capable of providing the best care possible.

8. Travelers

For frequent travelers, staying fit on the go can be a challenge. These 5-minute routines require minimal space and no special equipment, making them perfect for maintaining core strength and flexibility while traveling.

How to Use This Book

5-Minute core routines for seniors, 28-Day challenge with simple exercise to boost balance, lose weight and flexibility for healthy aging, this book is your guide to a healthier, more balanced, and flexible lifestyle, tailored specifically for seniors. Here's how you can make the most of it.

Getting Started

1. Understand the Layout: Each chapter in this book is designed to guide you through daily core exercises that can be completed in just five minutes. The 28-day challenge is structured to gradually build your strength and flexibility, ensuring that you progress safely and effectively.

2. Equipment and Preparation: The exercises in this book require minimal equipment. A comfortable mat, a sturdy chair, and a small set of hand weights are all you need. Ensure you have a dedicated, safe space where you can perform the exercises without interruptions.

Daily Routines

1. Follow the Daily Plan: Each day of the 28-day challenge has a specific set of exercises. Start with Day 1 and follow the routines in sequence, so try to perform the exercises at the same time each day to establish a habit.

2. Warm-Up and Cool Down: Begin each session with a gentle warm-up to prepare your body and reduce the risk of injury. Likewise, conclude each session with a cool-down routine to help your muscles recover and prevent stiffness.

Performing The Exercises

1. Clear Instructions: Each exercise comes with step-by-step instructions and a guide you are to follow. Pay close attention to the details of each movement to ensure you are performing them correctly and safely.

2. Modifications and Adaptations: We understand that everyone has different fitness levels and physical abilities. Each workout includes modifications to make it more accessible. If an exercise feels too challenging, start with the modified version and gradually work your way up.

3. Listening to Your Body: It's important to listen to your body and respect its limits. If you feel any pain or discomfort, stop right away and seek medical attention. The goal is to improve your strength and flexibility safely.

Staying Motivated

1. Track Your Progress: Celebrate your milestones, no matter how small, as they are indicators of your dedication and improvement.

2. Stay Positive: Maintain a positive mindset throughout the challenge. Remember that each step, no matter how small, is a move towards better health and well-being. Encourage yourself with positive affirmations and acknowledge your efforts.

3. Join a Community: Engage with others who are also on their fitness journey. Whether it's a local senior exercise group or an online community, sharing your experiences and progress can provide additional motivation and support.

Beyond The 28 Days

1. Maintain the Habit: Once you complete the 28-day challenge, continue incorporating these exercises into your daily routine. Consistent practice will help you maintain and further improve your balance, flexibility, and overall health.

2. Explore Further: Consider expanding your exercise procedure with other forms of physical activity that you enjoy. Activities like walking, swimming, or yoga can complement your core exercises and provide additional health benefits.

INTRODUCTION

It is my pleasure to Welcome to 5-Minute core routines for seniors, 28-Day challenge with simple exercise to boost balance, lose weight and flexibility for healthy aging."

As we age, maintaining our physical health becomes increasingly important. A strong core is essential for balance, stability, and overall mobility. It supports your back, improves posture, and makes everyday activities easier and more enjoyable. However, the idea of incorporating exercise into your daily routine can be daunting, especially if you're not used to working out regularly. That's why this book is here to help.

In the following pages, you will find a collection of easy-to-follow core exercises meant specifically for seniors. These routines are designed to be quick yet effective, ensuring you can fit them into your busy schedule without feeling overwhelmed. Each exercise focuses on strengthening your core muscles, enhancing your balance, and boosting your confidence in your physical abilities.

Remember, it's never too late to start taking care of your body. By dedicating just five minutes a day to these exercises, you'll be investing in your health and well-being. You'll soon notice improvements in your balance, strength, and confidence, empowering you to live a more active, fulfilling life.

Setting The Stage Embracing Healthy Aging

Aging is a process that brings wisdom and new experiences. Embracing these changes with a proactive mindset is crucial for maintaining an active and fulfilling life. This book is written in quest to navigating these changes through simple yet effective core exercises designed to boost balance and flexibility, helping you stay active, independent, and vibrant.

Symptoms and Causes of Balance Loss

Balance loss can present itself in various ways, such as:

Unsteadiness: Feeling wobbly or unstable while standing or walking.

Frequent Falls Experiencing more trips or falls than usual.

Dizziness or Vertigo: Sensations of spinning or light-headedness.

Difficulty with Daily Activities: Struggling with tasks that require balance, like climbing stairs or bending down.

Understanding the root causes of balance loss is essential. These can include:

Muscle Weakness: As we age, our muscles naturally lose strength, particularly in the core and legs.

Sensory Changes: Vision and inner ear changes can significantly affect balance.

Joint Stiffness: Arthritis and other conditions can lead to less flexible joints, making balance more challenging.

Neurological Issues: Conditions like Parkinson's disease and peripheral neuropathy impact coordination and balance.

Medications: Some medications have side effects that can impair balance.

What to Do When Experiencing Balance Loss

Experiencing balance issues can be concerning, but there are proactive steps you can take:

Consult a Healthcare Professional: Before starting any new exercise program, get a thorough check-up to rule out any underlying health issues.

1. **Gradual Progression:** Begin with simple exercises and slowly increase the intensity as you build strength and confidence.

2. **Use Support:** Incorporate supports like chairs, walls, or handrails to ensure safety during exercises.

3. **Consistent Practice:** Regular practice is key, to improving balance. Integrate exercises into your daily routine.

Important Questions to Ask

When dealing with balance loss, it's important to ask yourself and your healthcare provider the following questions:

When did you first notice your balance issues?

Are there specific activities or times of day when your balance is worse?

Have you had any recent changes in medication, diet, or health conditions?

Are there any other symptoms accompanying your balance issues, such as dizziness or vision problems?

What measures have you already taken to improve your balance, and what were the results?

Exploring Natural Remedies for Balance Loss

In addition to exercise, consider these natural remedies to support balance:

Balanced Diet

Ensure your diet is rich in vitamins and minerals, particularly Vitamin D calcium, and magnesium, which are vital for bone and muscle health.

Hydration

Dehydration can lead to dizziness and balance problems, so drink plenty of water.

Mindfulness Practices

Activities like yoga, Tai Chi, and meditation can improve balance by enhancing body awareness and reducing stress.

Herbal Supplements: Supplements like ginkgo biloba and omega-3 fatty acids may support brain health and improve balance.

CHAPTER ONE

UNDERSTANDING YOUR CORE

Your core muscles are the primary link in the chain that connects your upper and lower bodies. Several essential muscles work together to support and stabilize your motions.

Rectus Abdominis

The six-pack muscles run vertically down the front of your abdomen.

Transversus Abdominis

The deepest layer of abdominal muscles, which wraps around your sides and spine for support

Oblique

These muscles are usually found on the sides of the abdomen. They are classified into internal and external oblique's, which aid in twisting and bending actions.

Erector Spinae A set of muscles running down your spine that are essential for keeping an upright posture.

Pelvic Floor Muscles

These muscles provide support for your pelvic organs and help to maintain core stability.

Diaphragm

This major breathing muscle, located directly behind your lungs, also helps to maintain core stability.

Understanding these muscles and their functions is the first step toward efficiently strengthening your core.

Importance of Core Strength for Balance and Mobility

Your core muscles are engaged in practically every action you perform. They help you stand, sit, walk, bend, and even breathe. A strong core serves as a stable basis for all physical activity. Here's why core strength is important.

Balance: Core muscles help you stay balanced, reducing falls and boosting stability.

Mobility: A strong core allows for smoother, more efficient motions, simplifying daily chores easier.

Posture: Core strength is vital for excellent posture, lowering the risk of back discomfort, and maintaining a healthy spine.

Strength and Endurance

A strong core improves your total physical strength and endurance, allowing you to exercise for longer periods of time with less tiredness.

Benefits of a Strong Core

Building a strong core has various benefits, particularly as you age. Here are some of the main advantages.

Improved Balance and Stability

A strong core helps avoid falls by improving your balance.

Better Posture

Strengthening your core muscles promotes a healthier, more upright posture, which lowers the chance of back problems.

Enhanced Mobility

Core strength enables smoother and more efficient movement, making daily tasks easier.

Reduced Back Pain

A strong core can help to relieve and prevent lower back pain by supporting the spine.

Increased Confidence

Feeling steady and strong in your motions may increase your confidence in everyday tasks and social interactions.

How Aging Affects Balance and Core Strength

As we age, various variables might impair our balance and core strength

Muscle Loss

Age-related muscle loss, known as sarcopenia, can weaken core muscles, compromising stability.

Bone Density

Lower bone density can result in weaker bones, making falls more risky and recuperation more difficult.

Joint Stiffness

Arthritis and other disorders can cause less flexible joints, making balance more difficult.

Sensory Changes

Changes in vision, hearing, and proprioception (body position awareness) can all have an effect on balance.

Neurological Issues

Parkinson's disease and peripheral neuropathy affect coordination and balance.

Medications

Some medications have side effects that can impair balance.

Understanding these changes allows you to take proactive efforts to lessen their consequences, such as focused core workouts and balance training.

Self-Assessment Of Balance And Core Strength

Before beginning any new training plan, it is beneficial to evaluate your present balance and core strength. This self-assessment will serve as a benchmark for tracking your development and tailoring activities to your specific requirements.

Balance Assessment

1. **Single-Leg Stand:** Stand on one leg and maintain the posture for as long as possible. Note how long you can keep your equilibrium.

2. **Heel-to-Toe Walk:** Walk straight, with the heel of one foot squarely in front of the toes of the other. Count the number of steps you can take without wobbling.

3. **Chair Rise Test:** Sit on a chair and get up without using your hands. Count the number of times you can rise and sit in 30 seconds.

Core Strength Assessment

1. **Plank Hold:** Assume a plank position (on your elbows and toes) and hold the position for as long as possible. Record the time.

2. Leg Raise: Lie on your back, legs straight. Lift one leg to a 45-degree angle and hold for 10 seconds, then switch legs. Note any difficulty or discomfort.

3. **Seated Side Bends:** Sit in a chair with your feet flat on the floor. Bend sideways to each side, reaching your hand towards the floor. Notice any tightness or imbalance.

By understanding your current balance and core strength, you can better customize your exercise routine to address your specific needs and goals.

SUMMARY

In this chapter, we've explored the importance of the core muscles, their role in maintaining balance and mobility, the benefits of a strong core, and how aging affects these areas. We've also provided self-assessment tools to help you understand your starting point. With this foundation, you're ready to begin your journey towards improved balance and flexibility with the exercises and routines outlined in the following chapters. Remember, consistency is key, and every small step you take is a step towards a healthier, more active life.

CHAPTER TWO

PREPARING FOR EXERCISES

Creating a Safe Environment

Before starting any exercise routine, it's essential to ensure that your environment is safe and conducive to your workouts. Here are some steps to create a safe exercise space:

1. **Clear the Area:** Remove any obstacles, such as furniture, rugs, or clutter that could cause you to trip or fall.

2. **Non-Slip Surface:** Make sure the floor surface is non-slip. You might consider using a yoga mat or non-slip rug for added stability.

3. **Adequate Lighting:** Ensure your workout area is well-lit so you can see clearly and avoid accidents.

4. **Supportive Footwear:** Wear comfortable, supportive shoes that provide good traction and cushioning.

5. **Access to Support:** Have sturdy furniture or a wall nearby that you can use for support if needed during exercises.

6. **Stay Hydrated:** Keep water nearby to stay hydrated, especially during longer exercise sessions.

7. **Medical Clearance:** If you have any pre-existing health conditions, consult with your healthcare provider before starting a new exercise drill.

Importance Of Warm-Up

Warming up before exercising is very important to prepare your body for physical activity and prevent injuries. A proper warm-up gradually increases your heart rate, improves blood flow to your muscles, and enhances flexibility.

Gentle Warm-Up Routines

These are some gentle warm-up routines to get you started

1. **Marching in Place:** Begin by marching in place for 2-3 minutes, lifting your knees high and swinging your arms to gets your blood flowing.

2. **Arm Circles:** Stand with your feet shoulder-width apart and extend your arms out to the sides. Make little circles with your arms and gradually increase their size. Do this for 1-2 minutes in both directions.

3. **Side Steps:** Step side-to-side with your feet, gently swaying your arms. Continue this movement for 2-3 minutes to warm up your hips and legs.

4. Neck Rolls: To alleviate tension, gently roll your neck in a circular manner, first clockwise and then counterclockwise.

5. **Ankle Circles:** Lift one foot off the ground and make circles with your ankle. Do this for 30 seconds on each foot to warm up your ankles and feet.

Breathing Techniques for Effective Workouts

Proper breathing techniques can significantly enhance your workout performance and overall well-being. Here are some breathing techniques to incorporate into your exercises.

1. **Diaphragmatic Breathing:** it's known as belly breathing, this method includes inhaling deeply into your diaphragm rather than shallowly into your chest. Put one hand on your tummy, the other on your chest. Breathe in deeply through your nose, letting your stomach rise as you do. Exhale gently through your mouth, allowing your abdomen to descend. This technique helps engage your core muscles and improve oxygen flow.

2. **Pursed-Lip Breathing:** Inhale slowly through your nose and exhale through pursed lips, as if you are blowing out a candle. This technique helps regulate your breathing and maintain a steady pace during exercises.

3. **Coordinated Breathing:** Synchronize your breathing with your movements. For example, inhale during the preparatory phase of an exercise (such as lowering your body in a squat) and exhale during the exertion phase (such as standing up from the squat).

Visual Training for Vertigo

Vertigo and dizziness can be common issues, especially as we age. Visual training exercises can help improve your balance and reduce symptoms of vertigo.

1. **Seated Head Turns:** Sit comfortably in a chair and slowly turn your head from side to side, focusing your eyes on a specific point in the distance. Perform this exercise for 1-2 minutes.

2. **Standing Sway Shifts:** Stand with your feet shoulder-width apart and gently sway your body from side to side while keeping your eyes focused on a fixed point. Do this for 1-2 minutes to enhance your balance.

3. **Eye Tracking Movement:** Hold your thumb at arm's length in front of your face. Keep your head still and move your thumb up and down, side to side, while following it with your eyes. This exercise helps improve visual stability.

Dynamic Equilibrium Exercises

Dynamic equilibrium exercises involve movement and coordination, challenging your balance and core strength.

1. **Tandem Walking:** Walk in a straight line, placing one foot directly in front of the other, and heel to toe. To gain equilibrium, extend your arms out to the sides. Walk forward for 10-15 steps, then turn and walk back.

2. **Single-Leg Stand:** Stand on one leg with your other foot slightly off the ground. Hold this posture for 30 seconds and then swap legs. To make it more challenging, close your eyes or move your arms.

3. **Heel-to-Toe Walks:** Similar to tandem walking, but in a backward direction. This exercise enhances coordination and balance.

4. **Side Leg Rises:** Stand with your feet hip-width apart and lift one leg out to the side, keeping it straight. Hold for a few seconds and then start lowering it. Repeat 10-12 times on each side.

5. **Marching in Place with Head Turns:** March in place while turning your head slowly from side to side. This exercise challenges your balance by combining movement with head rotation.

SUMMARY

In this chapter, we've covered the essential steps to prepare for a safe and effective exercise routine. Creating a safe environment, warming up properly, practicing effective breathing techniques, and incorporating visual training and dynamic equilibrium exercises will help you maximize the benefits of your workouts. As you move forward, remember that consistency and gradual progression are key to achieving and maintaining better balance, flexibility, and overall health.

CHAPTER THREE

Seated Core Exercises

Seated core exercises are an excellent way to strengthen your abdominal muscles and improve stability while minimizing strain on your back and joints. Here are some effective seated core exercises:

Seated Head Turns

1. **How to Do It:** Sit comfortably on a chair with your feet flat on the floor. Slowly turn your head to the right, then to the left, keeping your shoulders relaxed.

2. **Benefits:** This exercise helps improve neck flexibility and can alleviate tension and stiffness.

Seated Leg Lifts

1. **How to Do It:** Sit on the edge of a chair with your hands gripping the sides for support Lift one leg straight in front of you, Hold the position for a few

seconds before gradually lowering it down. Repeat for the opposite leg. Repeat with the other leg.

2. **Benefits:** Strengthens your lower abdominal muscles and enhances leg strength.

Seated Spinal Twists

1. **How to Do It:** Sit upright on a chair with your feet flat on the floor. Position your right hand on the back of the chair and your left hand on your right thigh. Gently rotate your torso to the right, hold for a few seconds, and then return to the center." Repeat on the other side.

2. **Benefits:** Improves spinal flexibility and strengthens your oblique muscles.

Seated Core Twists with Belly Breaths

1. **How to Do It:** Sit on a chair with your feet flat on the floor. Place your hands on your knees. Inhale deeply, Inhale deeply, then exhale while turning

your torso to the right. Inhale as you return to the center, then exhale as you twist to the left.

2. **Benefits:** Enhances core strength and promotes deep, diaphragmatic breathing.

Seated Russian Twists

1. **How to Do It:** Sit on the edge of a chair with your feet flat on the floor and hands clasped together in front of you. Lean back slightly, keep your back straight. Rotate your torso to the right and then to the left while maintaining your core engaged.

2. **Benefits:** Strengthens the oblique muscles and improves rotational stability.

Seated Side Bends

1. **How to Do It:** Sit upright on a chair with your feet flat on the floor. Place your right hand on your right thigh and extend your left arm overhead. Bend your torso to the right, reaching your left arm over your head. Hold for a few seconds before

returning to the middle and repeating on the
opposite side.

2. **Benefits:** Stretches and strengthens the muscles
   along the sides of your torso.

Standing Core Exercises

Standing core exercises help improve balance and core strength by engaging multiple muscle groups simultaneously. Here are some effective standing core exercises:

Standing Sway Shifts

1. **How to Do It:** Stand with your feet shoulder-width apart. Shift your weight from one foot to the other, gently swaying your body side to side. Maintain control over your motions by engaging your core.

2. **Benefits:** Enhances balance and stability.

Marching in Place with Head Turns

1. **How to Do It:** Stand tall and march in place, lifting your knees high. While marching, turn your head slowly from side to side.

2. **Benefits:** Combines balance training with core engagement and improves coordination.

Single-Leg Stand with Knee Hug

1. **How to Do It:** Stand on one leg with your other knee lifted and hugged to your chest. Hold this stance for a few seconds before alternating legs.

2. **Benefits:** Strengthens the core and improves balance and stability.

Heel-to-Toe Side Steps

1. **How to Do It:** Stand with your feet together. Step to the side with your right foot, then bring your left foot to meet it, placing your heel to your toe. Repeat, moving to the left.

2. **Benefits:** Enhances balance and coordination.

Standing Pelvic Tilt with Torso Rotation

1. **How to Do It:** Stand with your feet hip-width apart. Tilt your pelvis forward and back to find a neutral position. From this position, rotate your torso to the right and then to the left.

2. **Benefits:** Strengthens the core and improves pelvic and spinal mobility.

Standing Oblique Crunches

1. **How to Do It:** Stand with your feet hip-width apart and hands behind your head. Raise your right knee to your right elbow while working your side muscles. Return to your starting position and repeat the maneuver on the left side.

2. **Benefits:** Targets the oblique muscles and enhances core stability.

Mat Exercises For Core Strength

Mat exercises are performed on the floor, providing a stable surface to engage your core muscles deeply. Here are some effective mat exercises:

Bird-Dog

1. **How to Do It:** Start on your hands and knees. Extend your right arm forward and your left leg back, keeping your back straight. Hold the posture for a few seconds, then move to the opposite side. "Is that clear?"

2. **Benefits:** Strengthens the core, back, and glutes while improving balance.

Plank with Chair Support

1. **How to Do It:** Place your hands on a chair and walk your feet back until your body forms a straight line from head to heels. Hold this position, keeping your core engaged.

2. **Benefits:** Strengthens the entire core and improves stability.

Lying Knee to Chest

How to Do It: Lie on your back with your knees bent. Be sure that one of your knees is up to your chest and hold on to it with your hands. maintain the position for some seconds. Change to other leg and repeat the process.

Benefits: Stretches the lower back and strengthens the lower abdominal muscles.

Lying Hip Bridges

1. **How to Do It:** concentrate as you Lie on your back with your knees bent and feet flat on the floor. Your hips have to be lifted towards the ceiling, make sure that squeez your glutes at the top. And after which lower your hips back down and repeat.

2. **Benefits:** Strengthens the glutes, hamstrings, and lower back.

Floor Leg Circles

1. **How to Do It:** Lie on your back with your legs extended. Lift one leg towards the ceiling and draw small circles with your foot. Perform in both directions, then switch legs.

2. **Benefits:** Strengthens the lower abdominal muscles and improves hip mobility.

Incorporating Weights for Added Resistance

Adding weights to your core exercises can help increase muscle strength and endurance. Here are some exercises incorporating weights:

Arm Chair Push-Ups

1. **How to Do It:** Sit on the edge of a chair with your hands on the armrests. Push yourself up slightly, then lower yourself back down. Use your arms to lift and lower your body.

2. **Benefits:** Strengthens the chest, shoulders, and triceps.

Seated Resistance Band Pulls

1. **How to Do It:** Sit on a chair with a resistance band looped around the legs of the chair. Hold the ends

of the band with both hands and pull them towards you, squeezing your shoulder blades together.

2. **Benefits:** Strengthens the upper back and shoulders.

Wall Push-Ups with Leg Raises

1. **How to Do It:** Stand facing a wall with your hands on the wall at shoulder height. Perform a push-up against the wall, and as you push back, lift one leg behind you. Alternate legs with each push-up.

2. **Benefits:** Engages the core and strengthens the chest, shoulders, and glutes.

Seated Resistance Band Leg Presses

1. **How to Do It:** Sit on a chair with a resistance band looped around your feet. Hold the ends of the band and press your feet forward, extending your legs. Return to the starting position and repeat.

2. **Benefits:** Strengthens the quadriceps and hip flexors.

Rotating Seated Leg Extensions

1. **How to Do It:** Sit on a chair with your hands on the sides for support. Lift one leg and extend it straight out in front of you. Rotate your leg in small circles, then switch legs.

2. **Benefits:** Strengthens the lower abdominal muscles and improves hip mobility.

Standing Calf Raises

1. **How to Do It:** Stand with your feet hip-width apart. Lift your heels off the ground, standing on your toes, then lower back down. For added resistance, hold a weight in each hand.

2. **Benefits:** Strengthens the calf muscles and improves balance.

SUMMARY

In this chapter, we've covered a comprehensive range of core exercises, including seated, standing, and mat exercises, as well as exercises incorporating weights for added resistance. These exercises are designed to enhance your core strength, balance, and flexibility, promoting overall health and mobility. Remember to perform each exercise with proper form and control, gradually increasing the intensity as your strength improves. Consistency is key to achieving and maintaining a strong, healthy core.

CHAPTER FOUR

BUILDING YOUR ROUTINE

Want to develop healthy new habits that will stick? While we occasionally succeed, we also face unexpected challenges. To avoid blockages and achieve our goals, we must establish and adhere to a new habit. Recognize that new routines might be tough.

Decide what needs to be in your routine.

Do you desire more exercise or more alone time? Prioritizing what is important to you before beginning is essential.

Set small goals.

Break down each huge aim into smaller ones. While a large objective is exhilarating to pursue, it frequently leads to failure because we take on too much. If your overall objective is to eat better meals, begin by changing one item each day to gain confidence. Congratulate yourself when you reach that goal.

Layout a plan.

Begin with one week at a time and work your way up to larger goals. Write it all down on a calendar, almost like an appointment.

Be consistent with time.

If you want to get in a daily walk, try doing it at the same time every day. Completing your chores first thing in the morning before you lose motivation helps you to reap rewards throughout the day. If you want to go to the gym, do it on your way to or from work; you will have better results. Most folks will not want to leave their cozy home once they arrive.

Be prepared.

When deciding on a new habit, make sure you have everything you need before you begin; this will make it simpler to get started right away. For example, if your new resolve is to clean the house every Saturday morning, ensure that your vacuum cleaner is in working order and that you have all of the necessary cleaning supplies.

Make it fun!

Getting into a new routine and new goals aren't always fun, but there are ways to make it fun. Find a workout buddy, get a good playlist for cleaning and try new cooking classes – anything to help you enjoy your new routine.

Track your progress.

Make a visual calendar where you may tick off each day you do the assignment. Most individuals do not want to "break the chain" and discover a blank area on their calendar.

Reward yourself.

Once you've created a steady pattern, treat yourself to something nice. For example, if your objective was to cultivate the habit of tidying up every night before bed, reward yourself with a new pair of slippers to wear around your newly cleaned house.

Exercises Around the House

1. **Squat While Brushing:** Squats may be performed while brushing your teeth or washing dishes by bending your knees and lowering your hips as if you were sitting in a chair. This strengthens your lower body and works your core.

2. **Wall Push-Ups:** During breaks or while waiting for something to cook, lean against a wall and do push-ups. This exercises the chest, shoulders, and arms.

Active Living Routines

1. **Take the Stairs:** Opt for stairs instead of elevators whenever possible. Climbing stairs is an excellent way to engage your leg muscles and core.

2. **Walk or Bike Short Distances:** Instead of driving for short trips, try walking or bicycling. This not only increases physical activity, but also improves mood and energy levels.

Managing Aches and Pains through Core Work

Core exercises play a vital role in managing and preventing aches and pains, especially in the lower back and hips. Here are some core exercises specifically designed for pain relief:

Seated Core Twists with Belly Breaths

1. **How to Do It:** Sit comfortably in a chair, feet flat on the floor, hands resting on your knees. Take a big breath in and exhale, twisting your torso to the right. Inhale as you return to the middle, then exhale and pivot to the left.

2. **Benefits:** Improves core strength and encourages deep, diaphragmatic breathing, which can help relieve stress and tension.

Seated Leg Lifts

1. **How to Do It:** Sit on the edge of a chair, hands clutching the edges for stability. Lift one leg straight out in front of you and hold for a few seconds before lowering it. Repeat with the other leg.

2. **Benefits:** Strengthens your lower abdominal muscles and improves hip mobility, reducing strain on the lower back.

Partner Workouts for Motivation and Accountability

Exercising with a partner can increase motivation and accountability, making your workouts more enjoyable and effective. Consider these partner exercises:

Partner Seated Resistance Band Pulls

1. **How to Do It:** Sit facing your partner with a resistance band looped around both of your feet. Hold the ends of the band and pull them towards you simultaneously, engaging your back muscles.

2. **Benefits:** Strengthens the upper back and shoulders while fostering teamwork and camaraderie.

Partner Standing Oblique Crunches

1. **How to Do It:** Stand facing your partner with your feet hip-width apart. Hold hands for stability and perform oblique crunches by lifting one knee towards the opposite elbow while twisting your torso. Alternate sides with each repetition.

2. **Benefits:** Targets the oblique muscles and improves core strength and coordination.

Flexibility and Posture Exercises

Maintaining good flexibility and posture is essential for overall health and mobility. Incorporate these exercises into your routine to enhance flexibility and posture:

Wall Angels

1. **How to Do It:** Stand with your back against a wall and your feet hip-width apart. Slowly raise your arms overhead, sliding them up the wall. Lower them back down, keeping your back and arms in contact with the wall throughout.

2. **Benefits:** Improves shoulder mobility, corrects rounded shoulders, and strengthens upper back muscles.

Chest Openers

1. **How to Do It:** Stand tall with your feet shoulder-width apart. Clasp your hands behind your back and gently lift your arms upward, opening your chest and stretching the front of your shoulders.

2. **Benefits:** Counteracts hunching and improves posture by opening up the chest and shoulders.

Cat-Cow Stretch

1. **How to Do It:** Start on your hands and knees in a tabletop position. As you inhale, arch your back and raise your head and tailbone to the ceiling, going into Cow Pose. Exhale as you round your back, tuck your chin to your chest, and tilt your pelvis under (Cat Pose). Alternate between the two poses in a flowing motion.

2. **Benefits:** Increases spinal flexibility, relieves tension in the back, and promotes better posture.

Forward Lean

1. How to Do It: Position your feet hip-width apart. Slowly bend at your hips and lean forward, maintaining a straight back and reaching for your toes. Hold the stretch for a few seconds, then return to the beginning position.

Benefits: Stretches the hamstrings and lower back, improving flexibility and posture.

Chin Tucks

1. **How to Do It:** Sit or stand tall with your shoulders relaxed. Gently tuck your chin towards your chest without tilting your head forward or backward. Hold the position for a few seconds, then release.

2. **Benefits:** Strengthens the muscles at the front of the neck, counteracting forward head posture and promoting better alignment.

SUMMARY

In this chapter, we've explored how to integrate core exercises into your daily routines, manage aches and pains through targeted workouts, incorporate partner exercises for motivation and accountability, and perform flexibility and posture exercises for overall well-being. By incorporating these exercises into your lifestyle, you'll not only strengthen your core but also improve your overall fitness, mobility, and quality of life. Remember to listen to your body, start carefully, and gradually increase the intensity and duration of your workouts for the best results.

CHAPTER FIVE

THE 28-DAY PROGRAM

We are glad that have you on board as you start your 28-Day Program, meticulously designed to boost your balance, flexibility, and overall core strength. This program offers a structured plan with daily exercises that gradually increase in intensity, ensuring a balanced and progressive approach to enhancing your physical well-being. Let's delve into the weekly breakdown, detailing the exercises and their benefits.

<h1 style="text-align:center">Weekly Breakdown</h1>

Week 1 Getting Started

Day 1: Gentle Warm-Up and Seated Head Turns

Gentle Warm-Up

Begin your workout with a 5-minute gentle warm-up to prepare your body for exercise. Light marching in place and arm circles will increase blood flow and loosen your muscles, reducing the risk of injury.

Seated Head Turns

Sit comfortably in a chair. Slowly turn your head to the right, hold for a second, and then turn to the left. This exercise helps improve neck flexibility and reduces stiffness. Perform 10 repetitions on each side.

Day 2: Seated Leg Lifts and Standing Sway Shifts

Seated Leg Lifts

Sit on the edge of a chair with your feet flat on the ground. Lift one leg at a time, holding each lift for a few seconds before lowering it back down. This exercise strengthens your quadriceps and hip flexors. Perform 10 lifts per leg.

Standing Sway Shifts

Stand with your feet hip-width apart and gently sway from side to side. This exercise enhances your balance and proprioception. Continue for 2 minutes, focusing on controlled movements.

Day 3: Seated Spinal Twists and Marching in Place with Head Turns

Seated Spinal Twists

Sit with your feet flat on the floor. Turn your torso to the right, hold for a few seconds, Rotate to the left. This exercise increases spinal mobility and improves digestion. Perform 10 twists on each side.

Marching in Place with Head Turns

March in place for 2 minutes, turning your head from side to side. This coordination exercise enhances balance and neck flexibility.

Day 4: Rest Day

Use this day to rest and recover. Rest days are crucial for muscle recovery and preventing overuse injuries. Stay hydrated and takes a gentle walk to keep your muscles loose.

Day 5: Seated Core Twists with Belly Breaths and Single-Leg Stand with Knee Hug

Seated Core Rotate with Belly Breaths

Sit on a chair and turn your torso to the right while exhaling deeply. Return to the center, you gently rotate to the left. This exercise engages your oblique muscles and promotes deep breathing. Perform 10 twists on each side.

Single-Leg Stand with Knee Hug

Stand and lift one knee to your chest, hugging it with both hands. Hold for 10 seconds and switch legs. This exercise improves balance and strengthens your core. Repeat 5 times per leg.

Day 6: Heel-to-Toe Side Steps and Seated Russian Twists

Heel-to-Toe Side Steps

Step sideways, placing the heel of one foot next to the toes of the other. This exercise challenges your balance and coordination. Repeat ten steps in either direction.

Seated Russian Twists

Sit with your knees bent and feet lifted off the ground. Rotate your torso to the right, to the left. This exercise strengthens your oblique muscles and improves rotational stability. Perform 10 twists on each side.

Day 7: Gentle Warm-Up and Seated Side Bends

Gentle Warm-Up

Repeat the warm-up routine from Day 1 to prepare your body for exercise.

Seated side bends sit comfortably, feet flat on the floor. Reach your right arm over your head and bend to the left. Return to the center and switch sides. This exercise stretches the side of your body and enhances flexibility. Perform 10 bends on each side.

Week 2: Building Strength

Day 8: Bird-Dog and Standing Pelvic Tilt with Torso Rotation

Bird-Dog

Start on all fours. Extend your right arm and left leg simultaneously, holding for a few seconds before switching sides. This workout strengthens your core and increases stability. Perform 10 reps per side.

Standing Pelvic Tilt with Torso Rotation

Stand with your feet hip-width apart. Tilt your pelvis forward and rotate your torso to the right, then to the left. This exercise engages your core and enhances flexibility. Perform 10 reps per side.

Day 9: Plank with Chair Support and Standing Oblique Crunches

Plank with Chair Support

Place your hands on a chair seat and extend your legs back into a plank position. Hold for 20-30 seconds, keeping your body in a straight line. This exercise strengthens your core, arms, and shoulders.

Standing Oblique Crunches

Stand with your feet shoulder-width apart. Lift your right knee towards your left elbow, engaging your oblique muscles. Switch sides and repeat for 10 reps each side.

Day 10: Lying Knee to Chest and Seated Resistance Band Pulls

Lying Knee to Chest

Lie on your back and bring one knee to your chest, holding it with both hands. This exercise stretches your lower back and hip muscles. Switch legs and repeat for 10 reps per side.

Seated Resistance Band Pulls

Sit with a resistance band looped around your feet, hold the ends and pull towards you, squeezing your shoulder blades together. This exercise helps to strengthen your upper back and shoulders. Perform 15 reps.

Day 11: Rest Day

Take a rest and let your body heal.

Use this time to relax and engage in light activities or gentle stretching to keep your muscles active.

Day 12: Arm Chair Push-Ups and Wall Push-Ups with Leg Raises

Arm Chair Push-Ups

Place your hands on the armrests of a chair, lower your body down, and push back up. This exercise strengthens your arms, chest, and shoulders. Perform 10 reps.

Wall Push-Ups with Leg Raises

Do a push-up against the wall, lifting one leg as you push back up. Alternate legs for 10 reps. This exercise enhances upper body strength and balance.

Day 13: Seated Resistance Band Leg Presses and Rotating Seated Leg Extensions

Seated Resistance Band Leg Presses

Sit with a resistance band around your feet and press your legs out against the band. This exercise strengthens your quadriceps and glutes. Perform 15 reps.

Rotating Seated Leg Extensions

Sit and lift one leg straight, rotating it outward and inward. This exercise targets your hip muscles and improves mobility. Perform 10 reps per leg.

Day 14: Standing Calf Raises and Floor Leg Circles

Standing Calf Raises

Stand with your feet hip-width apart, raise onto your toes, and lower back down. This exercise strengthens your calf muscles. Perform 15 reps.

Floor Leg Circles

Lie on your back, lift one leg, and make circular motions. This exercise strengthens your hip flexors and improves joint mobility. Perform 10 circles in each direction per leg.

Week 3: Increasing Flexibility

Day 15: Wall Angels and Chest Openers

Wall Angels

Stand with your back against a wall and move your arms up and down as if making snow angels. This exercise improves shoulder mobility and posture. Perform 10 reps.

Chest Openers

Clasp your hands behind your back, lift them slightly, and open your chest. This exercise stretches your chest and shoulders. Hold for 20 seconds.

Day 16: Cat-Cow Stretch and Forward Lean

Cat-Cow Stretch

Start on all fours, alternate between arching your back (Cow) and rounding it (Cat). This exercise improves spine flexibility and alleviates strain. Perform for 2 minutes.

Forward Lean

Stand and lean forward, reaching towards your toes, this exercise stretches your hamstrings and lower back. Hold for 20 seconds, repeat the exercise three times.

Day 17: Bird-Dog and Chin Tucks

Bird-Dog

Repeat the Bird-Dog exercise from Day 8 to continue building core strength and stability.

Chin Tucks

Sit or stand tall, gently tuck your chin towards your chest, and hold. This exercise strengthens your neck muscles and improves posture. Perform 10 reps.

Day 18: Rest Day

Use this day to rest and recuperate. Light activities or gentle stretching can help maintain flexibility and reduce muscle stiffness.

Day 19: Seated Core Twists with Belly Breaths and Plank with Chair Support

Seated Core Twists with Belly Breaths

Repeat the exercise from Week 1, Day 5, focusing on deep breathing and controlled movements.

Plank with Chair Support

Repeat the exercise from Day 9 to continue building core and upper body strength.

Day 20: Lying Knee to Chest and Heel-to-Toe Side Steps

Lying Knee to Chest

Repeat the exercise from Day 10 to maintain flexibility in your lower back and hips.

Heel-to-Toe Side Steps

Repeat the exercise from Week 1, Day 6, focusing on balance and coordination.

Day 21: Standing Pelvic Tilt with Torso Rotation and Seated Spinal Twists

Standing Pelvic Tilt with Torso Rotation

Repeat the exercise from Day 8 to enhance core strength and flexibility.

Seated Spinal Twists

Repeat the exercise from Week 1, Day 3 to maintain spinal mobility.

Week 4: Mastering Balance

Day 22: Seated Head Turns and Single-Leg Stand with Knee Hug

Seated Head Turns

Repeat the exercise from Week 1, Day 1, focusing on neck flexibility and relaxation.

Single-Leg Stand with Knee Hug

Repeat the exercise from Week 1, Day 5 to continue improving balance and core strength.

Day 23: Marching in Place with Head Turns and Standing Sway Shifts

Marching in Place with Head Turns

Repeat the exercise from Week 1, Day 3, enhancing coordination and balance.

Standing Sway Shifts

Repeat the exercise from Week 1, Day 2, focusing on balance and stability.

Day 24: Seated Russian Twists and Seated Side Bends

Seated Russian Twists

Repeat the exercise from Week 1, Day 6 to strengthen your obliques and rotational stability.

Seated Side Bends

Repeat the exercise from Week 1, Day 7 to maintain flexibility in your sides.

Day 25: Rest Day

Take a rest day to allow your body to recover. Engage in light activities or gentle stretching to stay active without overexertion.

Day 26: Arm Chair Push-Ups and Seated Resistance Band Leg Presses

Arm Chair Push-Ups

Repeat the exercise from Week 2, Day 12 to strengthen your arms and upper body.

Seated Resistance Band Leg Presses

Repeat the exercise from Week 2, Day 13 to maintain strength in your legs and glutes.

Day 27: Wall Push-Ups with Leg Raises and Rotating Seated Leg Extensions

Wall Push-Ups with Leg Raises

Repeat the exercise from Week 2, Day 12 to enhance upper body strength and balance.

Rotating Seated Leg Extensions

Repeat the exercise from Week 2, Day 13 to improve hip mobility and strength.

Day 28: Gentle Warm-Up and Standing Oblique Crunches

Gentle Warm-Up

Start with a gentle warm-up to prepare your body for the final exercise day.

Standing Oblique Crunches

Repeat the exercise from Week 2, Day 9 to finish the program with a focus on core strength and balance.

28-day program Conclusion

Congratulations on completing the 28-Day Program! By following this structured plan, you have taken significant steps toward improving your balance, flexibility, and core strength. Remember to maintain an active lifestyle and incorporate these exercises into your daily routine for long-term benefits. Celebrate your progress and continue embracing a healthier, more active life.

CHAPTER SIX

SUSTAINING YOUR PROGRESS

Integrating Core Exercises into Daily Habits

Integrating core exercises into your daily habits is essential for maintaining strength, balance, and overall health, especially as we age. By incorporating these exercises into routine activities, you can ensure consistency and reap the long-term benefits without dedicating separate time slots for workouts. Here's how you can seamlessly blend core exercises into your daily life.

Morning Routine

1. Stretch before Getting Out of Bed

Cat-Cow Stretch

While lying in bed, arch your back (Cow) and then round it (Cat). This gentle stretch awakens your spine and prepares your body for the day.

Knee to Chest

Pull one knee to your chest and hold for a few seconds, then switch legs. This exercise helps to relieve stress in your lower back.

2. Brushing Your Teeth

Standing Heel-to-Toe Stance

While brushing your teeth, stand with one foot directly in front of the other, heel to toe. This improves your balance and engages your core muscles.

3. Showering

Standing Side Bends

While in the shower, gently bend to each side, reaching your arm over your head. This stretches and strengthens your oblique muscles.

At Work

1. Sitting at Your Desk

Seated Spinal Twists

Sit upright and gently move your torso to the right, then to the left. This improves spinal mobility and reduces stiffness from prolonged sitting.

Seated Leg Lifts

Lift one leg at a time, holding for a few seconds before lowering. This strengthens your hip flexors and engages your lower abdominal muscles.

2. Taking Phone Calls

Standing March in Place

While on a call, stand up and march in place. This keeps you active, enhances your balance, and engages your core muscles.

3. Coffee Breaks

Standing Calf Raises

Stand with your feet hip-width apart, raise onto your toes, and lower back down. This strengthens your calf muscles and improves balance. Perform 10-15 reps during each break.

At Home

1. Cooking

Kitchen Counter Push-Ups

Place your hands on the edge of the counter and perform push-ups. This strengthens your upper body and core muscles. Aim for 10 reps while waiting for your food to cook.

Single-Leg Stands

Stand on one leg while chopping vegetables or stirring a pot. This enhances your balance and engages your core.

2. Watching TV

Seated Russian Twists

Sit on the edge of your couch, lift your feet slightly off the ground, and twist your torso from side to side. This exercise strengthens your oblique muscles.

Seated Core Twists with Belly Breaths

Sit upright and twist your torso to the right while exhaling deeply, then to the left. This engages your core and promotes deep breathing.

3. Household Chores

Vacuuming Lunges

As you vacuum, take a step forward into a lunge; bring your back leg forward. This strengthens your legs and engages your core muscles.

Laundry Squats

Squat down to pick up laundry or put it into the washer/dryer. This strengthens your legs and core.

Before Bed

1. Wind down Stretching

Forward Lean

Stand and gently lean forward, reaching for your toes. This stretches your hamstrings and lower back, promoting relaxation.

Wall Angels

Stand with your back against a wall, move your arms up and down as if making snow angels. This improves shoulder mobility and posture.

2. Deep Breathing Exercises

Belly Breaths: Sit or lie down comfortably. Place your hands on your abdomen, take deep breaths, and feel your belly rise and fall. This engages your diaphragm and promotes relaxation.

Tips for Success

1. Set Reminders

Use alarms or apps to remind you to perform these exercises throughout the day. Small, frequent sessions can add up to significant benefits.

2. Consistency is Key

Make these workouts a mandatory part of your everyday regimen. The more consistently you practice the more natural they will become.

3. Listen to Your Body

Pay attention to how your body feels. If any exercise causes discomfort or pain, modify or skip it. The goal is to enhance your well-being, not to strain your body.

4. Stay Hydrated

Drinking plenty of water throughout the day supports muscle function and overall health. Hydration is especially important when incorporating physical activity into your routine.

5. Enjoy the Process

Find joy in the small victories and improvements. Celebrating your progress, no matter how minor, will keep you motivated and committed to your health journey.

Tracking Your Progress: Before and After

Tracking Your Progress: Before and After

Tracking your progress is crucial to understanding how far you've come and staying motivated throughout your fitness journey. By documenting your starting point and monitoring improvements over time, you can celebrate your successes and make necessary adjustments to your routine. Here's a comprehensive guide to tracking your progress effectively.

Establishing Your Baseline

1. Initial Assessments

Body Measurements

Take measurements of your waist, hips, thighs, and arms. Use a flexible measuring tape and record the numbers accurately.

Weight: Weigh yourself using a reliable scale. Do this at the same time each day, preferably in the morning before eating or drinking anything.

Balance Tests

Perform simple balance tests such as standing on one leg or walking heel-to-toe in a straight line. Record how long you can maintain balance or how many steps you can take without losing stability.

Core Strength Tests

Perform exercises like planks or sit-ups and note how long you can hold a plank or how many sit-ups you can complete in a minute.

2. Photographic Evidence

Before Photos

Take clear, well-lit photos from the front, side, and back. Wear form-fitting clothing or similar outfits each time to easily compare changes over time.

3. Personal Reflections

Journaling

Write down how you feel physically and emotionally. Note any limitations or discomfort you experience in daily activities. Reflect on your energy levels, mood, and overall well-being.

Setting Realistic Goals

1. Short-Term Goals

Define your goals for the first month. Examples include improving balance, increasing flexibility, or enhancing core strength.

2. Long-Term Goals

Set goals for three, six, and twelve months. These could be more ambitious, like being able to perform more advanced exercises, achieving a specific weight, or significantly improving your posture and mobility.

3. Milestones

Break down your goals into manageable milestones. This could be weekly or bi-weekly targets that contribute to your short-term and long-term objectives.

Monitoring Progress

1. Weekly Check-Ins

Measurements and Weight

Record your body measurements and weight weekly. Look for trends rather than day-to-day changes.

Exercise Performance

Track the number of reps, duration, and intensity of your exercises. Note any improvements in balance, strength, or flexibility.

Photos

Take progress photos every two to four weeks. Compare them with your initial photos to visually assess changes.

2. Monthly Reviews

Reassessments

Perform the same balance and core strength tests you did initially. Compare the results to your baseline to see improvements.

Reflection

Write about any changes you've noticed in your physical abilities, energy levels, and overall well-being. Think about any problems you've experienced and how you overcome them.

3. Adjusting Your Plan

Exercise Routine

Based on your progress, adjust your exercise routine. Increase the difficulty or duration of your exercises as you become stronger and more balanced.

Goals

Revisit your goals and milestones. If you've achieved certain targets, set new ones to keep challenging yourself.

Celebrating Successes

1. Acknowledge Achievements

Celebrate reaching milestones and achieving your goals. This could be something simple like treating yourself to a favorite activity or sharing your progress with friends and family.

2. Reflect on the process

Take time to reflect on how far you've come. Re-read your initial journal entries and compare them with your current reflections to see the mental and emotional growth alongside the physical improvements.

3. Stay Motivated

Use your progress as motivation to keep going. Remind yourself of the positive changes you've experienced and the benefits of maintaining a healthy, active lifestyle.

Tools for Tracking

1. Fitness Apps

Utilize fitness apps that allow you to log your workouts, track your measurements, and monitor your progress. Many apps also offer reminders and motivational tips.

2. Wearable Devices

Consider using wearable fitness trackers to monitor your activity levels, heart rate, and even sleep patterns. These devices provide valuable data that can help you adjust your fitness plan.

3. Progress Journals

Keep a dedicated journal for your fitness journey. Record your measurements, photos, reflections, and milestones. This tangible record can be a powerful motivator.

Tips for Effective Tracking

1. Consistency is Key

Be consistent with your tracking methods. Measure and record progress at the same time of day and under similar conditions to ensure accuracy.

2. Be Patient

Understand that progress may be slow and gradual. Focus on the small improvements and trust the process.

3. Stay Positive

Maintain a positive mindset. Focus on what you have achieved rather than what you haven't. Celebrate modest wins and turn failures into learning opportunities.

By diligently tracking your progress before and after integrating core exercises into your routine, you'll have a clear picture of your achievements and areas for improvement. This not only keeps you motivated but also ensures that you're on the right path to healthier aging and a stronger, more balanced body.

Tips for Long-Term Maintenance and Improvement

Long-Term Maintenance and Improvement

Maintaining and improving your core strength, balance, and flexibility over the long term requires consistent effort, strategic planning, and a positive mindset. Here are some comprehensive tips to help you sustain and enhance your fitness journey:

Establishing a Sustainable Routine

1. Consistency Over Intensity

Regular Exercise

Commit to regular exercise rather than sporadic intense workouts. Most days of the week, aim to get in at least 30 minutes of physical activity.

Balanced Schedule: Create a balanced exercise schedule that includes core workouts, strength training, flexibility exercises, and aerobic activities.

2. Progressive Overload

Gradual Increase

Gradually increase the intensity, duration, and difficulty of your exercises to continue challenging your body and preventing plateaus.

Range

Use a range of workouts to target different muscle regions and avoid boredom.

3. Rest and Recovery

Scheduled Rest Days

Include rest days in your routine to allow your muscles to recover and prevent overuse injuries.

Active Recovery

Engage in light activities such as walking, stretching, or yoga on rest days to promote blood flow and recovery.

Setting Realistic and Achievable Goals

1. Short-Term and Long-Term Goals

SMART Goals

Set Specific, Measurable, Achievable, Relevant, and Time-bound (SMART) goals. This approach helps in creating clear and attainable objectives.

Milestones

Break down long-term goals into smaller milestones to stay motivated and track progress.

2. Personal Motivation

Intrinsic Motivation

Focus on intrinsic motivators such as feeling healthier, more energetic, and capable, rather than solely on external rewards.

Reward System

Establish a reward system for achieving milestones. Rewards can be non-food related, such as a massage, new workout gear, or a day off.

Embracing a Holistic Approach

1. Nutrition and Hydration

Balanced Diet

Consume a balanced diet rich in fruits, vegetables, lean proteins, whole grains, and healthy fats. Proper diet promotes muscle repair and general health.

Hydration

Stay well-hydrated by drinking plenty of water throughout the day. Dehydration can impair performance and recuperation.

2. Sleep and Stress Management

Quality Sleep

Aim for 7-9 hours of decent sleep every night. Sleep is crucial for muscle recovery, cognitive function, and overall well-being.

Stress Reduction

Incorporate stress management techniques such as meditation, deep breathing, and hobbies. Chronic stress can hinder progress and affect overall health.

3. Mental Health and Mindfulness

Positive outlook

Develop a positive mindset and engage in self-compassion. Recognize that failures are a part of the journey and use them as learning opportunities.

Mindful Practices

Engage in mindfulness practices such as yoga, tai chi, or meditation to enhance mental clarity and emotional balance.

Incorporating Functional and Everyday Activities

1. Functional Training

Daily Movements

Incorporate exercises that mimic daily movements to improve functional strength and make everyday activities easier.

Real-Life Scenarios

Practice lifting, bending, twisting, and reaching exercises that replicate real-life scenarios.

2. Active Lifestyle

Stay Active

Include physical activities in your everyday routine. Take the stairs, walk or bike for short trips, and engage in activities such as gardening or dancing.

Social Activities

Participate in group activities or sports that you enjoy. Social interaction can enhance motivation and adherence to an active lifestyle.

Regular Assessment and Adaptation

1. Periodic Assessments

Self-Evaluation

Regularly assess your progress through self-evaluation. Check your balance, flexibility, and core strength to identify areas for improvement.

Professional Assessment

Consider periodic assessments with a fitness professional to get expert insights and tailored recommendations.

2. Adaptation and Modification

Modify Exercises

Adapt and modify exercises as needed to suit your current fitness level, goals, and any physical limitations.

New Challenges

Introduce new challenges and variations to your routine to keep it interesting and to continue making progress.

Staying Informed and Educated

1. Continuous Learning

Education

Stay informed about new exercises, techniques, and fitness trends through books, articles, online courses, and fitness communities.

Expert Advice

Seek advice from fitness professionals, physiotherapists, or trainers to ensure you are performing exercises correctly and safely.

2. Staying Updated

Current Trends

Keep up with the latest research and trends in fitness and health to incorporate effective and evidence-based practices into your routine.

Networking

Join fitness groups or online forums to share experiences, gain insights, and stay motivated.

Cultivating a Support System

1. Accountability Partners

Workout Buddy

Find a workout buddy or join a fitness group to stay accountable and motivated. Exercising in groups may make exercises more pleasurable.

Community Support

Engage with online fitness communities or local groups for support, encouragement, and advice.

2. Professional Guidance

Personal Trainer

Consider working with a personal trainer for personalized guidance, motivation, and to ensure correct form and technique.

Health Professionals

Consult with health professionals such as dietitians, physiotherapists, or doctors to address any specific needs or concerns.

Conclusion: Your steps to Healthy Aging

As you reach the conclusion of this program, it's essential to reflect on the transformative journey you've undertaken toward healthy aging. The path to maintaining and improving core strength, balance, and flexibility is ongoing, but the rewards are profound and far-reaching.

Embracing a Lifelong Commitment

1. Consistency is Key

Daily Practice

The habits you've formed over the past 28 days are just the beginning. Consistency in your exercise routine is crucial for long-term health benefits. Continue to incorporate the exercises you've learned into your daily life.

Regular Review

Periodically review and adjust your routines to keep them challenging and effective. As your strength and balance improve, increase the intensity or complexity of your workouts.

2. Holistic Approach

Balanced Lifestyle

Healthy aging isn't just about physical activity. A balanced approach includes proper nutrition, adequate sleep, stress management, and mental wellness. Ensure that all these aspects are integrated into your daily life.

Mindfulness

Practice mindfulness and positive thinking. A good thinking has a tremendous influence on your motivation and general well-being. Celebrate your progress and acknowledge the effort you've put into your health.

Reaping the Benefits

1. Physical Well-being

Improved Mobility

Enhanced core strength and balance lead to better mobility and reduced risk of falls. You'll find daily activities, such as walking, bending, and lifting, easier and more comfortable.

Pain Management

Regular core exercises can help alleviate common aches and pains, particularly in the lower back. Flexibility exercises can reduce stiffness and improve joint health.

2. Mental and Emotional Health

Increased Confidence

As you gain physical strength and stability, your confidence in your abilities will grow. This can positively impact other areas of your life, including social interactions and mental health.

Stress Reduction

Physical activity has been shown to help reduce stress. Regular exercise can help manage anxiety and depression, promoting a more relaxed and happy state of mind.

3. Social Connections

Community Involvement

Engaging in group exercises or community fitness programs can foster social connections. Building relationships with others who share similar goals can provide support and motivation.

Family Participation

Encourage family members to join you in your exercise routine. It can be a fun and healthy way to spend quality time together and promote healthy habits for everyone.

Looking Ahead

1. Setting Future Goals

New Challenges

As you become more comfortable with your current routine, set new goals to keep pushing your limits. Consider trying new activities or sports that interest you.

Personal Milestones

Set personal milestones for ongoing improvement. These could be related to weight, strength, balance, or overall fitness levels.

2. Lifelong Learning

Stay Informed

Keep up with the latest research and trends in fitness and health. Staying informed will help you make better decisions and continue to improve your routines.

Seek Expertise Don't hesitate to seek advice from fitness professionals, dietitians, or physiotherapists to optimize your exercise regimen and address any specific needs or concerns.

3. Adaptability

Listen to Your Body

Observe how your body reacts to various workouts. Adapt and modify your routines as needed to prevent injury and ensure they remain effective.

Be Flexible

Life can be unpredictable, and maintaining flexibility in your approach to exercise is essential. If you miss a day, do not be disheartened. Get back on track and continue your journey.

Final Thoughts

Your journey to healthy aging is a testament to your commitment to improving your quality of life. The progress you've made is commendable, and the habits you've developed will serve you well in the years to come. Remember, healthy aging is a continuous process that requires dedication and a positive attitude.

Reflecting on Achievements and Transformations

As you approach the culmination of your 28-day journey, it's time to pause and reflect on the significant strides you've made. This period of introspection is not just about acknowledging the physical changes but also about recognizing the emotional and mental transformations you've experienced. Each step, each exercise, and each moment of perseverance has led you to this point. Embrace the fullness of your achievements and the profound impact they have on your life.

Embracing Physical Progress

1. Increased Strength and Stability

Core Strength

Feel the newfound power in your core muscles. The once-challenging exercises now come with a sense of ease and control. Your core strength has improved, providing a solid foundation for your overall physical health.

Enhanced Balance

Notice how your balance has become more reliable. Daily activities like walking, climbing stairs, and even standing still are now performed with greater confidence and stability. The fear of falling has diminished, replaced by a sense of security and self-assurance.

2. Flexibility and Mobility

Greater Flexibility

Appreciate the increase in your range of motion. The flexibility exercises have eased stiffness and made movements more fluid. Whether reaching for something high or bending down, you move with greater grace and comfort.

Improved Mobility

Celebrate the ease with which you now navigate your world. Improved mobility means more independence and freedom to enjoy life without physical limitations holding you back.

Mental and Emotional Triumphs

1. Building Confidence

Overcoming Challenges

Reflect on the obstacles you have overcome. Each time you pushed through a tough workout or completed a challenging routine, you proved to yourself that you are capable and resilient. This confidence extends beyond exercise, enriching other areas of your life.

Positive Self-Image

Your self-perception has transformed. The dedication and hard work have not only improved your physical appearance but also how you see yourself. You carry yourself with pride knowing that you have invested in your well-being.

2. Emotional Well-Being

Stress Reduction

Remember the days when stress weighed heavily on your shoulders. Regular physical activity has lightened that burden. The exercises have become a sanctuary, a time to release tension and find peace within you.

Emotional Resilience

Your emotional resilience has strengthened. The commitment to your health has fostered a sense of accomplishment and a positive outlook. You've learned to face challenges with a calm mind and a steady heart.

Celebrating Personal Milestones

1. Small Wins and Big Victories

Daily Achievements

Each day brought small victories – completing an extra rep, holding a pose longer, or simply showing up. These daily achievements add up, creating a powerful momentum that drives you forward.

Significant Milestones

Reflect on the major milestones – the day you first balanced on one leg without wobbling, the moment you realized your back pain had eased, or the time you completed a full routine without feeling exhausted, these are not just physical triumphs but symbols of your dedication and progress.

2. Personal Transformation

Physical Changes

Look in the mirror and see the physical changes. Notice the toned muscles, the improved posture and the vitality in your step. These visible transformations are the result of your hard work and commitment.

Inner Growth

Beyond the physical, recognize the inner growth. You have developed discipline, perseverance, and a deep sense of self-worth. The journey has shaped you into a stronger, more resilient, and more confident individual.

Moving Forward with Gratitude

1. Gratitude for the Journey

Acknowledging Efforts

Be grateful for the effort you have put in. Each drop of sweat, each moment of determination, and each instance of pushing through discomfort has been worth it. Your journey is a testament to your strength and resolve.

Appreciating Support

Recognize the support you've received from family, friends, or even yourself. The encouragement and motivation have played a crucial role in your success.

2. Looking to the Future

Continued Commitment Let this process be the foundation for continued growth. Stay committed to your health and well-being, use the skills and habits you've developed to maintain and further your progress.

Inspiring Others

Your transformation can inspire others. Share your journey, motivate those around you, and be a beacon of what dedication and hard work can achieve.

Final Reflections

As you reflect on your achievements and transformations, take a moment to be proud of how far you've come. This journey is not just about physical changes but also about discovering your inner strength and potential. You have proven that with dedication, perseverance, and a positive mindset, you can achieve great things.

Encouragement for Continued Wellness

Dear Reader,

As you near the end of this life transformative adventure, I want to offer words of encouragement for your continued wellness. Your dedication to improving your core strength, balance, and flexibility has been inspiring, and I believe that with persistence and a positive mindset, you can maintain and even enhance your well-being in the days ahead.

Embracing a Lifestyle of Health

1. Consistency is Key

Daily Practice

Keep up with your daily exercises. Consistency is the cornerstone of continued progress. Even on days when motivation wanes, remind yourself of how far you've come and the benefits you've experienced.

Routine Check-ins

Regularly assess your routines. Are they still challenging enough? Do you need to modify or add new exercises? Adjustments ensure that your workouts remain effective and engaging.

2. Holistic Wellness

Nutrition

Remember that exercise is just one part of a healthy lifestyle. Pay attention to your nutrition, ensuring you fuel your body with nourishing foods that support your fitness goals.

Rest and Recovery

Do not underestimate the value of rest and recovery. Allow your body time to heal and recharge between workouts. Quality sleep is essential for overall well-being.

Nurturing Mental Resilience

1. Mindful Practices

Mindfulness Meditation

Incorporate mindfulness techniques into your daily life. Meditation, deep breathing exercises, or mindful movement can help reduce stress, improve focus, and enhance your overall mental well-being.

Positive Affirmations

Practice positive self-talk. Affirmations such as "I am strong and capable" or "I am committed to my health" can reinforce your dedication and motivation.

2. Stress Management

Stress-Relieving Activities

Find activities that help you unwind and destress. Whether it's reading, listening to music, spending time in nature, or pursuing a hobby, prioritize activities that promote relaxation and joy.

Seek Support

Don't hesitate to reach out for support if you're feeling overwhelmed. Talk to friends, family, or a mental health professional if you need guidance or a listening ear.

Setting Goals and Staying Motivated

1. Goal Setting

Define Objectives

Set clear, achievable goals for your wellness journey. Whether it's increasing workout intensity, improving flexibility, or mastering new exercises, having specific targets keeps you focused and motivated.

Celebrate Milestones

Milestones should be celebrated as they represent your growth. Recognize and praise yourself for accomplishing any milestone, no matter how tiny. Each achievement is a step forward in your wellness journey.

2. Stay Inspired

Inspiring Resources

Surround yourself with inspiring content. Read books, listen to podcasts, or follow social media accounts that promote health, fitness, and positivity. Inspiration can come from various sources.

Community Engagement

Join a group of people who share your beliefs. Join fitness classes, online forums, or social groups where you can share experiences, seek advice, and find encouragement.

Embracing Change and Adaptation

1. Flexibility in Approach

Adapt to Challenges

Life is full of ups and downs. Be adaptable and resilient in the face of challenges. If circumstances change or obstacles arise, adjust your plans and strategies without losing sight of your goals.

Explore Variety

Keep your wellness journey exciting by exploring new activities or variations of exercises. Variety not only prevents boredom but also challenges different muscle groups and keeps your body responsive.

2. Listen to Your Body

Body Awareness

Tune in to your body's signals. Be aware of any pain, discomfort, or exhaustion during your workouts. Take rests as needed to avoid overexertion. Your well-being is a priority.

Final Words of Encouragement

Your commitment to wellness is a testament to your strength and resilience. Remember that wellness is a journey rather than a destination. Accept each day with a feeling of purpose and drive. You have the power to create a life filled with vitality, joy, and continued wellness.

May you find inspiration in your achievements, strength in your challenges, and fulfillment in your journey towards a healthier, happier you.

Looking Ahead to a Stronger, More Flexible Future

I want to take a moment to look ahead with you. The progress you've made, the challenges you've overcome, and the dedication you've shown are all stepping stones toward a stronger, more flexible future. Let's envision what lies ahead and how you can continue to thrive in the days to come.

Cultivating Strength and Resilience

1. Building Physical Strength

Progressive Training

Continue to challenge yourself with progressive exercises. Gradually increase the intensity, duration, or complexity of your workouts to keep pushing your physical limits and building strength.

Functional Fitness

Focus on exercises that enhance your functional fitness movements that mimic activities of daily living. This approach not only strengthens muscles but also improves coordination and balance in real-world scenarios.

2. Enhancing Flexibility

Dynamic Stretching

Incorporate dynamic stretching into your routine to improve flexibility and range of motion. Dynamic stretches involve moving parts of your body through a full range of motion, helping to prevent injury and enhance performance.

Yoga and Mobility Work

Explore yoga or mobility-focused workouts. These practices not only increase flexibility but also promote relaxation, mindfulness, and a deeper connection between mind and body.

Setting New Goals and Challenges

1. Pushing Boundaries

Goal Setting

Define new goals that align with your evolving fitness journey. Whether it's mastering advanced yoga poses, increasing resistance in strength training, or participating in a fitness event, set targets that excite and motivate you.

Cross-Training

Consider cross-training to add variety and challenge to your workouts. Incorporate activities like swimming, cycling, hiking, or dance classes to engage different muscle groups and prevent plateaus.

2. Embracing Versatility

Functional Movements

Focus on functional movements that enhance everyday activities. Squats, lunges, pushes, pulls, and twists strengthen not just isolated muscles but entire movement patterns crucial for functional fitness.

Mind-Body Connection

Explore mind-body practices such as tai chi, Pilates, or meditation. These disciplines not only improve physical well-being but also cultivate mental clarity, focus, and emotional balance.

Nurturing Holistic Wellness

1. Prioritizing Recovery

Rest and Regeneration

Embrace the importance of rest days and recovery strategies. Allow your body time to heal and regenerate, optimizing performance and reducing the risk of overuse injuries.

Sleep Quality

Maintain healthy sleep habits. Quality sleep is essential for recovery, hormone regulation, cognitive function, and overall well-being. Create a sleep-friendly environment and prioritize sufficient rest each night.

2. Mindful Nutrition

Balanced Diet

Continue to nourish your body with a balanced and nutrient-rich diet. Prioritize whole foods, plenty of fruits and vegetables, lean proteins, healthy fats, and adequate hydration. Fueling your body optimally supports your fitness endeavors.

Embracing a Lifelong Journey

1. Lifelong Learning

Educational Pursuits

Stay curious and open to learning. Explore workshops, courses, or seminars related to fitness, nutrition, mindfulness, or holistic wellness. Continuous learning enhances your knowledge base and empowers you to make informed choices.

Self-Reflection

Take time for self-reflection and introspection. Assess your progress, celebrate achievements, learn from setbacks, and adjust goals as needed. Self-awareness is an effective technique for personal development.

2. Community and Support

Engage with Others

Stay connected with a supportive community. Surround yourself with others who share your enthusiasm for wellbeing. Participate in group activities, seek advice, offer encouragement, and celebrate successes together.

Resources

These are some valuable resources to support your ongoing learning and growth. These resources encompass additional tools, recommended reading materials, and a handy index for quick navigation, ensuring you have access to comprehensive guidance and information.

Additional Tools and Materials

1. **Fitness Apps and Online Platforms:**

Explore fitness apps and online platforms that offer workout routines, tracking features, and educational content. Examples include fitness trackers, yoga apps, meditation guides, and nutrition planners.

2. **Home Exercise Equipment:**

Consider investing in home exercise equipment that complements your fitness goals. Options may include resistance bands, dumbbells, stability balls, yoga mats, foam rollers, and balance boards.

3. Workshop and Training Programs:

Attend workshops, seminars, or training programs focused on specific aspects of wellness, such as strength training, flexibility, mindfulness, nutrition, or injury prevention.

4. Educational Videos and Tutorials

Access online videos and tutorials that demonstrate proper exercise techniques, stretching routines, meditation practices, and wellness strategies, quality instructional content can enhance your understanding and execution of fitness principles.

Recommended Reading and References

1. **Wellness and Fitness Books:**

Explore books on wellness, fitness, nutrition, and mindfulness written by experts in the field. These books offer valuable insights, practical tips, and evidence-based strategies for optimizing health and well-being.

2. **Scientific Journals and Research Papers**

Delve into scientific journals and research papers related to exercise physiology, biomechanics, aging, balance training, flexibility enhancement, and other relevant topics. Stay informed about the latest advancements in wellness science.

3. **Nutrition Guides and Cookbooks**

Consult nutrition guides and cookbooks that emphasize healthy eating habits, balanced meals, nutrient-rich recipes, and dietary strategies to support fitness goals and overall wellness.

Index for Quick Navigation

1. Organized Content

Utilize the index for quick access to specific topics, exercises, techniques, and resources mentioned throughout this book. The index serves as a navigational tool to help you find information efficiently.

2. Key Concepts and Terminology

Refer to the index for definitions of key terms, concepts, and principles discussed in the chapters. Enhance your understanding by exploring related topics and cross-referencing relevant content.

Bonus: Seated Sun Salutation

let's explore the Seated Sun Salutation an adaptation of the traditional yoga sequence designed to promote flexibility, mindfulness, and overall well-being. Whether you're new to yoga or seeking a seated variation for comfort and accessibility, the Seated Sun Salutation offers a gentle yet invigorating practice to uplift your mind, body, and spirit.

Seated Sun Salutation Steps

1. Begin in a Comfortable Seated Position:

Sit tall on a chair or mat with your spine straight and shoulders relaxed. Place your hands on your knees or thighs, palms facing down or up as desired.

2. Inhale: Mountain Pose (Urdhva Hastasana):

As you inhale, raise your arms overhead, reaching towards the sky. Keep your shoulders relaxed, lengthen your spine, and engage your core gently.

3. Exhale: Forward Fold (Uttanasana)

On the exhale, slowly hinge forward from your hips, bringing your chest towards your thighs. Let your hands rest on the floor, legs, or ankles, depending on your flexibility.

4. Inhale: Half Lift (Ardha Uttanasana)

Lift your torso slightly, lengthening your spine and reaching forward. Keep your back flat, gaze forward, and engage your abdominal muscles for support.

5. Exhale: Seated Forward Bend (Paschimottanasana)

Release deeper into the stretch as you fold forward from your hips, aiming to bring your chest closer to your thighs, relax your neck and shoulders, allowing gravity to deepen the stretch.

6. Inhale: Reverse Half Lift (Ardha Uttanasana Variation)

Lift your torso halfway, extending your arms forward or placing your hands on your shins. Lengthen your spine, open your chest, and draw your shoulder blades together.

7. Exhale: Return to Mountain Pose (Urdhva Hastasana)

Slowly rise back up to the starting position, bringing your arms overhead with palms facing each other. Feel the stretch through your sides and spine as you reach upward.

Benefits of Seated Sun Salutation

Improved Flexibility

The sequence gently stretches the spine, hamstrings, and shoulders, promoting flexibility and mobility.

Mind-Body Connection

Focus on mindful breathing and movement coordination to enhance awareness and relaxation.

Energizing and Uplifting

The flow of the sequence can invigorate your energy while calming your mind, leaving you feeling refreshed and centered.

Accessible and Comfortable

Suitable for all fitness levels and can be done seated, making it accessible for individuals with mobility limitations or those seeking a gentle practice.

About This Book

This book is a comprehensive guide to improving balance and flexibility through targeted core exercises. It is designed for seniors and those looking to maintain or regain their balance and mobility. Each chapter provides detailed instructions and tips for exercises that can be performed at home, with minimal equipment. The 28-day challenge offers a structured program to help you steadily progress and see real improvements.